Chakras For Beginners

*Ultimate Guide To Understanding The Power of Chakras For Beginners.*

**By Karen Hunt**

# Chapter 9 - Using the Power of Affirmations to Balance Your Chakras

## Your Chakra Journey

## Introduction to Chakras

Welcome to my book called *"Chakras for beginners"*, and inside I'm going to share with you how understand chakras can improve your life and wellbeing 100%

It's really about connecting your true mind, body and spirit using the natural phenomenon of our energy chakras.

I actually first learned about chakras around 10 years ago when a friend of mine who had discovered about his chakras years before started to show me the benefits of chakras and meditation.

Every since that day I've been hooked and fascinated by chakras and so I've decided to know reveal to you the proven steps and strategies on how to quickly and easily learn the benefits of chakras and how to use them effectively along with the seven key important chakras.

This book is a perfect read if you want to get started with learning the true benefits of understanding your chakras.

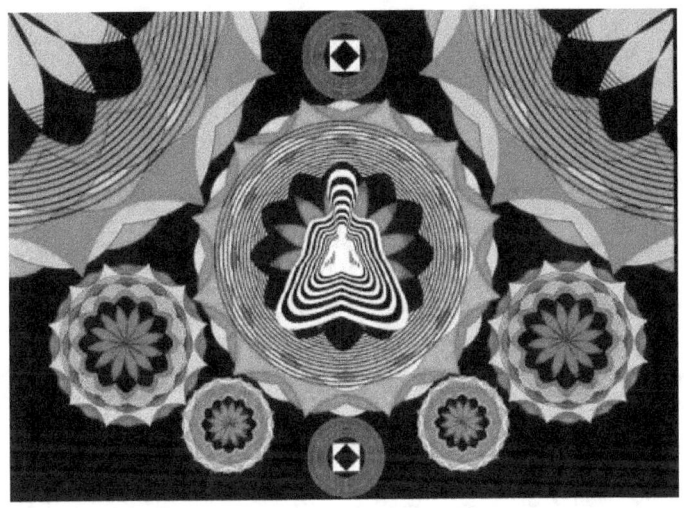

# Chapter 1: Understanding Chakras

If you find yourself trapped inside the confinement of our modern existence and feel far from your true self, it's time to embrace some ancient eastern spirituality. Exploring the unknown territories where your body, mind and soul converge can be a life altering journey.

The concept of chakra originates from tantric and yogic traditions of Hinduism and Buddhism. The word chakra means "wheel" in Sanskrit and promotes the idea of constant cyclic movement around a center (hub). The best way to describe a chakra is to imagine a colorful wheel or flower that undergoes permanent spinning. The chakra colors are the same you can see in the rainbow; red, orange, yellow, green, blue, indigo, and violet and each chakra is stimulated by its own and complementary color.

It is important to acknowledge that these are not organs, or physical parts of your body, but more like nodes of concentrated energy, able to radiate to a certain extent. If the chakras are not balanced well enough, the overall condition of a person has to suffer. It is important to understand the concept of energetic balance and how to achieve it. Too much or too less energy can have equally negative effects on all levels of someone's existence. The body experiences fatigue, disease, injury, while the mind develops negative thoughts and emotions. Life quality and the possibility to be happy are seriously endangered. On the other hand, a constant balance between the chakras promotes health and a sense of well being, which in turn help an individual become successful and enjoy life.

As a fact, normal people are not able to see chakras but those claiming to be clairvoyants describe them as colorful light emitted by the subjects, proportional to their energy levels. The existence of chakras has yet to be proven by scientist, but there is a least a shred of evidence to the entire story. Any object that has a temperature above absolute 0 emits radiation, some of which takes the form of light. The human body is actually bioluminescent, but to such a small degree that our eyes are not able to see that faint light. You are probably familiar with the term "aura"

There are many chakras mapped along the human body, but only seven are considered to be most important. The seven chakras begin at the top of the head (crown chakra) and end at the base of the spine (root chakra).

## Chapter 2: First Chakra

The root chakra, called Muladhara, is associated with the color red and is symbolized by a yellow, square lotus, surrounded by eight shining spears on the sides and with four red petals at each of its corners. This energetic center is located at the base of the spine between the tailbone and the pubic bone. The position inside the human body means that the root chakra governs over the legs, hips and sexual organs.

At the physical level, Muladhara controls and influences sexuality, a big component of every individual's well being. After all, the archetype of making sure our genes are transmitted to future descendants is a major concern during our entire life. Muladhara refers mostly to masculine sexuality, and this is because a man's sexual organs are located near its hypothetical centre.

At the mental level, Muladhara is connected with stability and the ability of an individual to develop a mentality for life. Muladhara is associated with the element of earth, the sense of smell and the action of excretion. Because it is associated with the sense of smell, it is also associated with the nose, and because it is associated with excretion, it is also associated with the anus.

Being the lowest of all chakras, many people consider it inferior and not worth working upon. In fact, Muladhara is the foundation of the entire energy body and who would want to build anything on a week foundation? Many interpretations over the role of each chakra tend to consider the root chakra the essential building block and the most easy to improve.

It is considered that imbalances of the root are responsible for inducing anemia, fatigue, lower back pain, and even depression. The root can be stimulated with intense physical exercise and restful sleep. Anything red increases the energy of this chakra.

## Chapter 3: Second Chakra

The second chakra, also called Swadhisthana, is symbolized by a lotus that encircles a crescent moon, with six orange petals on the outside. Alternative names for it are the belly, sacral chakra, or spleen chakra. The name Swadhisthana can be traduced from Sanskrit as "one's own abode".

This energetic centre of the body controls mainly the emotional part of human behavior, with creativity, friendliness, confidence, joy, enthusiasm and sense of self-worth being directly linked with the stimulation at this level. Because women's sexual organs are located primarily in the second chakra, Swadhisthana is linked with female sexuality, focused more on the emotion level than on the physical level.

If enough energy flows through the second chakra, the individual is able to be an integer part of his/her social environment and to express emotions about himself and the others. If somehow energy is not able to each this point, then the individual will feel hold back from living a normal and satisfactory life inside society. Obsessions, emotional instability and a chaotic or unfulfilled sexual life are all symptoms of problems with the sacral chakra. More aggravated forms include violence and addictions.

Imbalances of this chakra are responsible for eating disorders, alcohol and drug abuse, back pains, allergies and urinary problems. Malfunctions of the libido like impotency and frigidity are also regarded as direct effects of an inefficient sacral chakra.

Being the second chakra, Swadhisthana is associated with orange, the second color of the light spectrum. Thus, activity in this region is stimulated by orange food and drinks. You can also increase its energy levels by practicing water aerobics or by receiving massage.

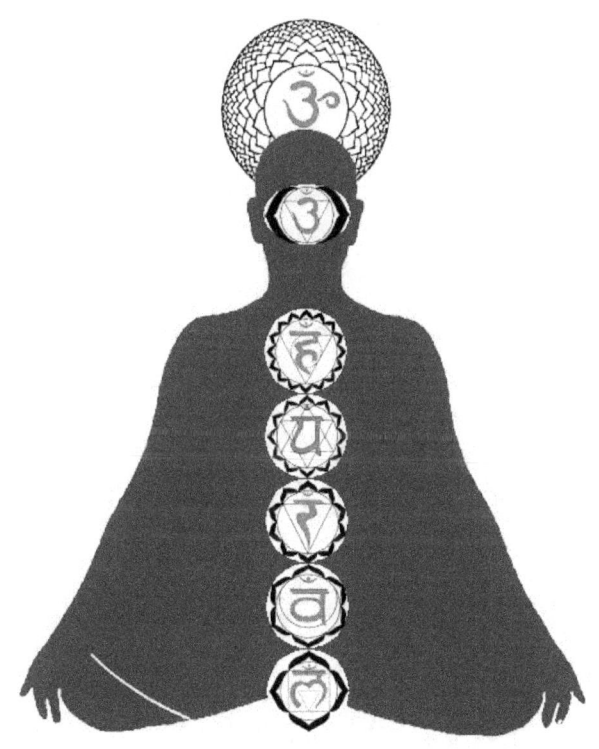

## Chapter 4: Third Chakra

Moving up in the body, the third chakra, also called Manipura, is represented as a triangle pointing down, circumscribed by a circle with ten petals along its exterior. The color associated with this Manipura is yellow, so anything matching the color, from food to clothes, is able to help increase energy levels or remove existing blockage.

The Manipura is located between the sternum (breastbone) and the stomach and is also referred to as the solar plexus. This position means that it is able to directly influence the digestive system, and even metabolism. The importance of this chakra is highlighted by the fact that at its level the body obtains energy from the digested food. Any disturbances are reflected in the body's poor capacity of using the external resources, thus limiting the ability to heal and replace damaged cells. Physical problems revolve around all sorts of digestive problems, among which ulcers, liver problems, constipation, parasites, colitis, food allergies, abnormal high or low sugar levels in the blood are the most frequent. As a side fact, Manipura was traced down with accuracy inside the human body and it is believed that it resides in a group of pancreatic cells called Islets of Langerhans.

The third chakra is unanimously looked as the center of personal power, the place from which the ego is inflated, and all kind of explosive emotions are released. Anything driven by passion, impulse or anger is loaded with energy received from Manipura. Individuals with high levels of such energy, unable to drain it to other chakras, usually experience nervousness and irritability. These states usually evolve to full-scale uncontrollable outbreaks of fury, usually directed towards the others, that leave the body in a state of nervous exhaustion. Lack of confidence, confusion, even depression can seriously impair one's life. Restoring balance at this level brings back self-respect, the desire to accept new challenges, making that person more cheerful and outgoing

## Chapter 5 – Fourth Chakra

Anahata, the fourth chakra of the human body, is also called the heart chakra. The complexity of its symbol follows the same ascendant path, and it is built from a hexagram (two intersecting triangles, symbolizing the union between male and female) and an exterior circle with twelve green petals.

Anahata is related to green, so anything of this color is able to increase the energy flow at this level of the body. Being placed in the center of the chest, near the heart, any imbalances are able to inflict heart and breathing disorders, like high blood pressure, chest pain, heart attacks. The proximity to the thymus means that any imbalance also affects the immune system, the body's defensive mechanism. After all, heart diseases are the most common causes of death. Thus it is crucial to look after this chakra with maximum care and satisfy its energetic demands. The best ways to do that are taking extended walks in nature, as well as spending time with friends and family. Eliminating major sources of stress is another key to assure that your Anahata is working properly.

At the emotional level, the heart chakra is what drives you to be compassionate, friendly, and empathetic with the others. It is what we sum up as kind. The desire to see what's good in everything and everyone, to always choose to see the full half of the glass, comes from deep inside the fourth chakra. Probably most import, the feeling of love, the supreme feeling a human being is capable of producing, originates here. Balance means an individual is equally equipped for giving and receiving love, the same way energy flow to and from any chakra in the human body. If few resources are available, and those few resources are captured by negative emotions and worrying thoughts, there are slim chances for love to occur. Love is a pyramidal construction, and its foundations are self acceptance, forgiveness and compassion.

As we see, the structure and functionality of whole system of chakras allocates inferior levels for pure sexuality and a higher one for love. This does not mean one is less important than the other. If you put them on a scale, they are equally important, but directing energy to the higher levels requires much more effort. It is somehow similar to the pressure required for water to climb up a pipe. The higher it needs to go, the higher the imposed pressure must be.

Tibetan Buddhism sees in Anahata the home of the indestructible red/white drop, responsible for transporting our consciousness to the next life. If you believe in reincarnation and eternal life lived in different bodies, this presence teaches you that the body is more than just a vehicle. At least a part of it is immortal and transcends from one existence to another. That hope makes justice to

an old Latin phrase: Finis vitae sed non amoris -
"The end of Life is not the end of Love".

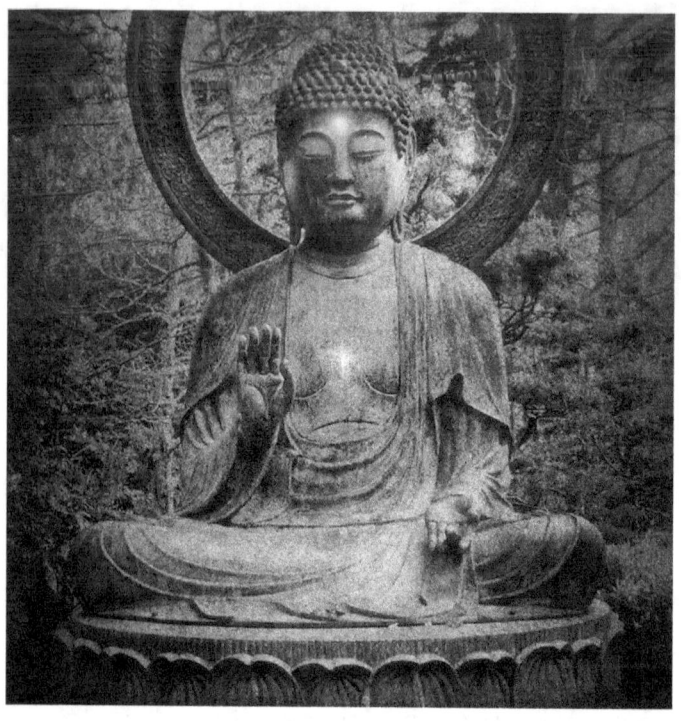

## Chapter 6 – Fifth Chakra

The fifth chakra, called Viduddha in Sanskrit, is located in the throat region, marking the advance of the chakra system towards the upper limit of the body, the head. The symbol of the fifth chakra is composed of a downward triangle, which both includes and is included in adjacent circles. The exterior circle is decorated with sixteen turquoise petals.

Color blue, the fifth color of the spectrum of visible light, holds a strong connection with the throat chakra. Any form of blue in your daily life is able to boost this energetic centre and make it converge to a level of balance.

The Viduddha is strongly connected with the body's main channels of communication. The voice is produced by the larynx, an organ included in the influence area of the fifth chakra. Physical effects of imbalance include all kinds of infections, disorders linked to the way hormones are released in the body, hyperactivity and any kind of problems regarding mouth, jaw, tongue or neck. The affected area can stretch as far as the shoulders.

The fifth chakra is able to influence how a person embraces change, transformations and personal healing. One's ability to communicate and express itself in a natural and efficient manner is dictated by energy being stored and released in Viduddha. You can recognize individuals with imbalance at this level by the way they act and speak. Holding back thoughts, having a quiet voice or simply being unable to communicate with the others are all major signs of concern. People who achieved full control over energy flow at this chakra benefit from extended concentration, creativity, ease of expression and artistically perspective.

Singing, engaging in fruitful conversations or sustaining meaningful speeches are all means to exercise the "muscle" of the throat chakra.

## Chapter 7 – Sixth Chakra

Approaching the end of the chakra ladder, we find Anja, also called the third eye, or brow chakra. Located just above the eyes, in the center of the forehead, this chakra symbolizes clairvoyance and a higher understanding of things. The center exerts control over the brain, face, eyes and endocrine system

As the symbols for higher end chakras are becoming more and more complex, Anja takes a few steps back, being represented only by a lotus with two petals. Simplicity evokes an approach that reduces everything to its essence, to its core values, closer to the greater truth. Indigo is the color associated with the sixth chakra, so any contact with objects, clothes or food of this color empowers the centre to collect, store and use more energy from the outside.

Anja is also the point where the two parallel nadis (Ida and Pingala) merge with the central channel Sushumna, marking the end of duality in the chakra system. The road is set for the ultimate chakra to be reached.

Carefully planned sessions of meditation are able to stimulate the activity of the sixth chakra. Like stated before, higher chakras are less accessible for most of the humans, due to their position. If not looked after and controlled, energy is more prone to stay on lower levels. It is the same behavior shared by all objects attracted by gravity – the search for low potential, easy to maintain positions.

Anja is all about looking beyond reason and trusting your intuition and insight. The third eye becomes open and a new perspective over the world enters the stage. Keeping that eye open means trusting inner guidance at any step of the way. The road you are walking on is a path of enlightenment, which will eventually take you to your higher self. It was reported that telepathy and powerful hallucinations involving travels in other planes of existence came along for those able to perfectly tune Anja.

At this level, a precarious balance can favor learning disabilities, lack of coordination and sleep disorders. Even more disastrous, you could lack initiative and actually be afraid of having success. The prospect of becoming something else, even though we are talking about a better person, is felt as scary and dangerous. Opening the third eye is a painful experience for a chakra which is not able to feed on enough energy. Other physical symptoms may include vision deficiencies and headaches.

## Chapter 8 – Seventh Chakra

Lastly, we will talk about the seventh chakra, Sahasrara, also named the crown chakra, which is located just behind the top of the skull. The name reflects the fact that it holds the highest position in the chakra hierarchy, marking the center of spirituality and enlightenment. This is our bridge with divinity and here takes shape what we like to call God. It is assumed that this is the portal used by the soul when it enters or leaves the body.

Translated from Sanskrit, the name Sahasrara means a lotus with one thousand petals. This is also the symbol used to portray the chakra. In Tibetan Buddhism it takes the form of a white circle, with 33 downward pointing petals.

There are two colors usually associated with the crown chakra. First there is purple, the end color of the light spectrum, and the second one is white, symbol of completeness (if we mix all colors of the light spectrum we obtain a white beam of light).

Sahasrara, in its balanced form, can be a level of pure consciousness, in which all links with the material (mortal) world are cut. Even the death of the body does not represent a concern, because the elevated inner self can now access eternity. The conscious and subconscious are merging to form something beyond human understanding. This high energy arrangement of the chakras inside the human (also called karma body) is very unlike to be achieved by most humans during their lifetime.

Many mysterious medical conditions like mental illness and epilepsy are regarded as disturbances of energy levels at the level of the seventh chakra (possible long phase variations).

## Chapter 9 - Using the Power of Affirmations to Balance Your Chakras

Informing yourself about chakras is not enough to get a taste of their true potential. Here you can find a compilation of apparently simple affirmations that will charge you with energy at all the 7 levels.

1. I am a harmonious human being and I feel peaceful and protected.

2. I am happy, confident, and strong and I enjoy the life I live.

3. I have complete control over my life and I am succesful. My life is full of rewards.

4. Love is the solution for everything and I shall bring love in this world.

5. I am free to think only at the truth and express my true thoughts.

6. I understand and accept everything because everything was revealed to me.

7. I am complete. I am one with the Supreme Being I believe in.

Repeat them as many times you want and feel free to search for others or write down your very own versions. The recipe for writing good affirmations is to concentrate only on the positive things you want to have in your life. Use as many favorable adjectives and adverbs, but keep the phrase sounding natural.

It is a proven fact that repeating to yourself a phrase, the meaning of the words actually reaches your subconscious and directs your actions towards a certain purpose. After all, ideas become words, and words written down soon become actions. If you repeat something many times, it will also be written in your mind.

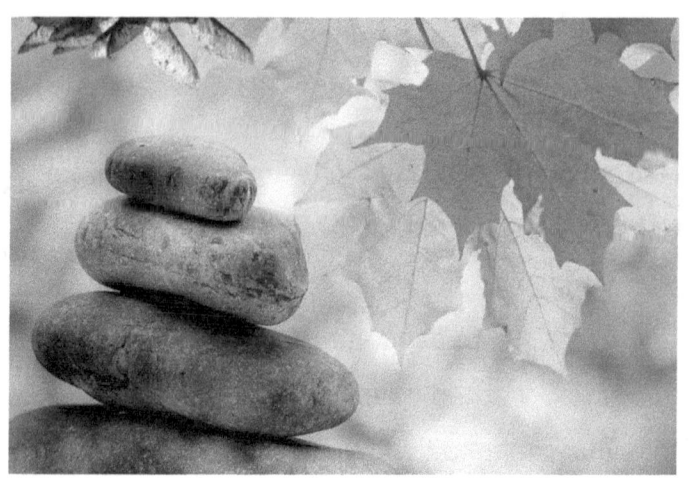

## Your Chakra Journey

Thank you again for downloading my book on chakras.

I hope this book gave you a true understanding of what chakras really are and how you can use all seven chakras to help improve your life and live it to the fullest and happiest.

The next step is to take action on what you have learned today.

Finally, if you enjoyed this book, then I'd like to ask you for a favor, would you be kind enough to leave a review for this book on Amazon? It'd be greatly appreciated as it helps more people like yourself find my book and spreads the positive message on helping more people reap the benefits of understanding their chakras.

Thank you and best wishes,

Karen Hunt

I have decided to add 2 bonus books I've wrote that I thought you might like on Auras and Reiki healing.

# Auras

## *Beginners Guide To Seeing, Hearing and Feeling Auras.*

## By Kathy Hunt

Introduction

What is an Aura?

How Do You See Auras?

The Kirlian effect

The Direct Meaning of Auras and Their Colors.

The Red Aura

The Orange Aura

The Yellow Aura

The Green Aura

Soft Blue Aura

Black Auras

A White Light Aura

Conclusion On Your Aura Journey

**Introduction**

Welcome to this beginners guide on auras where you will discover how to see, sense and feel auras in your daily life.

Auras really are amazing when you have your first experience them, you will be never forget it!

I've wrote this short book in an easy to understand format so that you can easily apply what you learn fast all about auras.

Keep an open mind and enjoy the spiritual journey.

Kathy Hunt

What is an Aura?

In today's time, extended access to information and scientific research had left little room for superstition and the unknown.

We want to see evidence before we accept something as being true. But there are still dark corners of our current understanding of the world, places where phenomenon we haven't manage to explain still survive, feeding our belief that we have many things to explore before claiming to posses full knowledge. What we consider paranormal is just the limit of knowledge and we put this label to anything beyond our reach.

We should not fear the unknown, but cultivate a desire to explore.

An aura is defined to be a subtle luminous radiation, surrounding a person and generated by energetic fields that travel throughout the body.

Auras have yet to be confirmed by mainstream science, but there are numerous arguments to support the claim that we are talking about a real phenomenon. It is said that all living things (including humans) and all objects manifest such an aura, which for some is more prominent and easy to observe.

Auras has been associated with spirituality and religion and depictions of deities and holy persons usually portrait them with extended auras.

In religious art, auras can be identified as a halo or aureola surrounding the head or the entire body. From Christianity to Buddhism and in every other major religion, the existence of aura is accepted as a fact and the more visible and extended the light is, the more holly is that particular figure inside the religious hierarchy. Auras with extended magnitude, visible for the eye of the uninitiated are those belonging to holly men.

A possible explanation for the aura phenomenon comes from medical science. The theory claims that auras are ghost images generated by malfunctions of the brain or of the visual system.

Conditions like epilepsy, migraines or the effect of psychedelic drugs are all responsible for altering the way reality is experienced trough the senses. Although it seems convincing enough, it is dangerous to accept such a local explanation as the general truth.

Another breakthrough in explaining why some people are convinced they are seeing auras is the identification of a neuropsychological phenomenon called emotional synesthesia.

In a few words, the areas in the brain responsible for processing stimuli from the senses are intensely interconnected.

You could easily call it a cross-wiring that renders errors. Thus reality is perceived in a modified, maybe enhance form.

From this point of view, color synestheshia means that the brain region responsible for face recognition is associated with the color-processing region.

Psychic abilities to observe aura emanations had been tested, but with inconsistent results. One such test involves asking the psychic to count the number of persons in a dark room based on the number of auras he/she could observe.

Another test required psychics to distinguish between real persons and mannequins hidden behind opaque partitions. The only conclusions from these test was that many people claim to poses psychic abilities.

Like with any other controversial subject, we have the two sides that throw arguments one at each other. For a neutral observer, new to the subject in matter, choosing what truth to believe and what side to support can be a hard decision. Beyond all claims, belief is something we feel from inside and it is beyond our control.

Can we imagine a world where we take for real only what we directly experience?

Could we trust each other if we claim solid evidence for everything? So the question "Is the auras real?" is wrongly formulated. A more correct approach would be: "Am I ready to accept that there are things beyond my reach and my knowledge about the world is limited?"

We can point out as being completely truth the fact that, like any other object that has a temperature above 0 degrees, the human body generates heat and a small dose of luminous radiation. The body definitely has a weak electromagnetic field surrounding it and that field varies in intensity depending on how active we are. The light we see and perceived as being white can be broke in his building blocks, the colors of the spectrum.

## How Do You See Auras?

Modern medicine, still limited to the traditional way of healing just the body and neglecting the true sources of disease, was not able to encourage the development of technology capable of showing auras.

Anyone interested in maintaining a healthy aura today must rely on others capable of seeing or sensing life energies. It is a matter of trust to take for granted what you are not seeing with your own eyes, but you have little to lose.

We all fear to believe things because we fear the disappointment of investing energy in something that isn't there.

The best reason to believe in auras is the fact that placebo medicine has prove to have strong roots in reality. What we chose to believe can actually influence real world events so the form of energy we are after is hidden somewhere for sure.

In order to be able to see auras you have to open your mind in order to learn about them. When the time is right, all your preparation will prove its usefulness and you will truly see auras.

Human senses are closely connected one to each other. Some people develop what is called as synesthesia, a mix of senses which would confuse most of us. Such an experience can be that of tasting or smelling colors with science being unable to fully explain how and why it occurs.

Continuing the idea, you need to sense first the auras, by collecting information from all the possible sources, in this case, all the senses the human body was gifted with. That means paying attention how you feel near someone's presence. Don't focus on the body language, but more on the impression that individual is producing to you. Ask yourself how you feel when you are alone and how you feel with that particular person. A good advice is to use someone you are neutral to instead of choosing someone able to generate strong emotions.

Color coding is very useful even in the early stages. It is useful to use the same correspondence described in the next chapter in order to get used with what each color of the aura means.

Learning to see auras is very much related to optics.

It is recommended to develop the ability to extend your field of view beyond its normal limit because thus you activate cells on the retina which are more sensitive to light. Concentration exercises are also very useful.

As you will look at one object at a time you will be able to spot subtle tones and many details your superficial normal sight don't usually allow.

You will later need to obtain higher and higher levels of concentration if you plan to be able to see auras.

Pay attention to colors, especially those of natural origin. Observe how the quantity and orientation of light changes how we see colors and details.

Train your eyes to see colors in the dark. Close your eyes and try to guess what colors different objects around you have. Ask someone to help you in this initiative and take things very seriously.

Practice is the key for training your eyes to see auras but you will need also to train your mind.

Read as much as possible about the whole phenomenology behind the visible spectrum of light. The light is your field of study now so it's perfectly natural to ask yourself all kind of questions about light.

You could begin by exploring why the sky turns red at sunset or why a clear sky at noon looks blue. Study natural phenomena similar to auras, like rainbow or the Glory or any other atmospheric occurrence involving light.

If you want to be sure you are on the right track, asking for professional advice from a credible person who claims to be able to read auras is the best thing you could do. There are secret techniques you probably won't find on the Internet and for a good reason.

Who would give away its tools of the trade for free? If you like more the scientific approach, joining optic classes or renting a laboratory to test your assumptions is even better. Reach out and you will find many others like you, who are convinced that auras are there to be seen.

A fear of ridicule prevents many from continuing to believe, but if you are not afraid to stand behind what you believe than you will have made the hardest step.

## The Kirlian effect

One alleged way of seeing someone's aura is by what is called the Kirlian effect. Kirlian photography is a collection of photographic techniques used to capture the phenomenon of electrical coronal discharges.

It was noticed that from person to person, the impressions of the auras varied. The idea states that their images showed a life force or energy field generated by the body and in direct relation with the physical and emotional states of their living subjects.

It is important to acknowledge that by reading the aura it becomes possible
to diagnose malfunctions in the body (diseases) long before physical symptoms take shape and induce pain and suffering. Also, at your limited level of experience reading auras the best you can achieve is to detect what intentions people have regarding you.

It means going beyond the limits of intuition and trying to figure out is someone is lying to you or faking a smile.

It is a huge social advantage to be able to read people and many successful professionals owe their career to having a better understanding of how others think and act.

## The Direct Meaning of Auras and Their Colors.

Beyond all definitions, the aura is our bodies output of energy. Being of electromagnetic nature it can be associated with a range of colors.

The same we see light in different colors throughout the Universe based on its wave length, a meaning for aura color can be extracted.

Any known color to the human eye can also be retrieved by reading someone's aura. Dependencies can be established between the ideas, feelings and level of health a person is experiencing and the colors found in his/her aura.

Sometimes things can be confusing because the same color can be used to give opposite readings, but there is a coherence a seasoned reader will understood.

Tonality of colors has an easy to understand key. As we will further see, dark colors present in aura readings are usually considered to be reflections of negative feelings of thoughts, obstructions for the energy flow.

## The Red Aura

Red is the color we usually associate with blood, the heart, circulation and thus the human body from the anatomical point of view.

It is a natural assumption to make that the presence of red, amongst others colors signals vitally and life in its prime. But red can also be tied with experiencing intense emotions. Clear red, the red we know as traditional red denotes a powerful, passionate and competitive individual.

Strong sexuality could also be associated with this kind of red. Pink and more subtle shades of red are signs of love, romantic relationships or feelings of affection and tenderness.

Higher sensitivity and a more artistic nature can also be unearth by observing auras with a bright and more pale red. Dark red is generally considered to be a sign of dormant anger ready to emerge.

The energetic individual becomes violent as its red part of the aura becomes darker and darker.

Dark tones of pink are signs of immaturity and dishonesty.

Individuals dominated by red aura color share robust personalities enjoying the physical aspects of life. They live their lives in the present with almost infinite resources of strength, stamina, courage, and self-confidence.

They are usually hard working and pro-active and are the ones in search for immediate results.

In a conversation with someone dominated by red you will immediately spot honesty and to the point phrases. The approach can indeed be to direct and personal, but this is a mark that makes them popular and successful.

In fewer words, reds are those who enjoy and welcome life and take their roles to the fullest extent.

## The Orange Aura

Orange is a mix from red and yellow so it's very likely that you'll see influences from the characteristics associated with those colors.

In terms of the psychical body, orange is usually reserved to the reproductive system, so if readings identify some auras dominated by orange we are dealing with highly sexual active individuals.

Personalities governed by orange live with a tremendous inflow of energy, both physical and mental. They are very tuned in with the environment and are able to adapt to new scenarios with unmatched ease.

Overcoming obstacles at work or in relationships and high endurance are also marks of the presence of this color in the aura output. The high energy levels are sometimes hard to control, so individuals experience exuberance and excess. Sensibility to addictions is present trough their lives and short explosive episodes occur.

The approach to relationships is usually full of lust and passion. The shift towards yellow means we are dealing with creative, intelligent and detail oriented person. The scientific way is the one of choices for auras dominated by this color.

### The Yellow Aura

Moving on to yellow, this is the color strictly associated with life energy flowing trough and out of the body.

When the color dominates the aura spectrum we are talking about someone who is well connected to life and anything around him. A bright, attention-grabbing color, yellow creates a sensation of brightness and warmth similar to that you experience in a summer day.

The color attracts those looking for joy, light and comfort. It can be noticed that more people are drawn to a person emanating yellow light than normal. If you have a yellow aura, it means that you are a very generous person and that you are open in sharing everything you know or poses with the others around.

If this is the case, you are a messenger of love and hope to those you come in contact with. Light yellow indicates some sort of awakening to a greater truth or a struck of genius regarding an idea.

Extreme optimism and unbeaten hope are also expected from someone emanating such an aura. Moving on, shiny metallic gold yellow is a sign that awakening or revelation is building up to reveal a greater truth and energy levels are at their maximum. We are probably talking with someone very special who might become a very important public figure.

Gold is a universal symbol for rarity and high value and the same can be said about someone who develops gold like kind of aura.

Dark yellow can be read from a person obsessed or preoccupied with an activity that drives him/her over the limits, without meaningful results.

Fatigue and stress can be guessed only by seeing that muddy yellow light leaving the body. Yellow resembling lemons, marks other imbalances in one's behavior and spiritual state. It is usually encountered at individuals who are afraid of losing something (a material possession, statute, power, or someone loved). Clinging too much to something we are probably not meant to have drains too much energy from body in a way that is undesirable. With this leakage there, that individual will gradually lose touch with other aspects of life and find itself in dead end.

**The Green Aura**

With green we are reaching for a more cooler and easy to watch color of the spectrum.

We traditionally associate green with nature, ecology, rebirth and fertility. Watching something green makes us feel more optimists and take things easy. From the start, reading of green in the aura output of energy indicates we are dealing with someone who is a natural healer.

Using words or simple actions they are able to relief negative feelings and take things of your chest.

They can inspire change and evolution to a higher mental and physical state or simply help those around achieve peace of mind and balance.

A special kind of green, that similar to mint leaves is a strong indicator we are dealing with a very spiritual person. Sometimes that potential is hidden behind layers and layers of other colors and only someone experienced can see that faint presence. Apple green Is also associated with healing, but shifts mostly towards healers of the human body.

Care takers, medics and often parents develop in their energetic output such a shade of green, which can be traduced as a focus towards making someone else feel good. Although it may be though so, light green is not something desirable within someone's aura. That person might develop a very efficient way of promoting disappointment around and also getting away with it. Shimmering green is a mark of healers of another kind.

They are those around us able to interact to everyone and are a pleasure to be around in almost every social situation. They steal the show, take center stage, know the best jokes and give the best reply. Looking at green in general, it is a comfortable color to be around and you get the instant feel of growth, balance and time efficiently spent.

Beside medics, teachers with love for their job present the same chromatic dominance. Like wit the other colors present inside an aura, dark tones of green are signs of flaws or deficiencies.

Muddy green is usually translated as sensitivity towards criticism and a very easy to break ego.

Low self-esteem is also present together with that tonal output.

As you probably guessed, the next color we are talking about, blue, is a mark of cold and distance, and lacks the turbulent nature and high energetic of other colors.

Soft Blue Aura

Soft blue identified in readings of the aura indicates we have in front a highly intuitive, intelligent, devoted and caring personality. Soft light blue indicates a state of peace, clarity in the thought process and unmatched open attitude towards communication.

You can always trust a person dominated by blue light as it will have few reasons to lie or take advantage. Some abilities of clairvoyance and an elevated spiritual state can be linked with intense blue.

Finding the right way in life and having all things sorted out are also attributes able to generate blue light in the outside world. Like most of the darker tones, we can also feel the presence of fear inside dark flat blue. It is usually the fear which projects future outcomes in a negative manner and could be considered the opposite of an optimistic attitude.

An individual unable to express itself or who experiences restraints in the way of being honest about his/her problems will have the aura dominated by the same shift towards darker blue.

Indigo marks few individuals and is a sign that the third eye is about to open and a different understanding of the world is about to be embraced by the mind. High sensitivity and unmatched intuition powers.

Indigo light is reserved for a limited number of people to be able to produce and is a clear sign we are dealing with someone special.

The final light of the color spectrum, also find in aura readings is associated with the nervous system and extended mental abilities.

High levels of intuition, fertile imagination and visionary episodes produce an output of violet light, making the aura complete.

Beside the seven main colors, there are other colors or non-colors that deserve special attention.

**Black Auras**

Black is characteristic for bodies which work very well in attracting and absorbing energy. Black presence inside the aura means that the individual is struggling with unresolved issues that are preventing him/her to go one about one's life. Light of any other colors is darkened by the presence of black and the joy of living can be considered hijacked by a side goal. In most of the cases that goal is a negative one, like revenge, but there are cases when the human is able to reduce energy flow to a minimum in order to redirect it one channel only.

Healing from a life threatening condition can render the aura reading to be dominated by black as the body is reestablishing what was close of losing.

## A White Light Aura

A white light often represents a new, not yet designated energy in the aura.

White light is a strong indicator of pregnancy and marks the birth of a new energy source. Pastels, sensitive blends of light and color are able to highlight an unusual sensitivity and a need for serenity throughout expression. Artists are those to display such colors in the aura.

Grey, brown and anything in between are signs of blocked energies. The individual governed by such aura lights is stagnant in his/her evolution and goes through life without getting involved too much in it and without enjoying what he/she does..

## Conclusion On Your Aura Journey

So now I have taken you on a journey into the world of auras, I really hope this book will help you to see, sense and feel auras.

The next step is to take action on what you have learned today.

Like I mentioned at the beginning of this book, seeing and feeling auras is an amazing experience that words can't always describe but make sure you feel free to share what you have learned with your family and friends.

Finally, if you enjoyed this book, then I'd like to ask you for a favor, would you be kind enough to leave a review for this book on Amazon? It'd be greatly appreciated!

Enjoy your journey,

Karen Hunt

# Reiki For Beginners

## Discover The Ancient Methods Of Reiki Healing

By Karen Hunt

## Introduction

Welcome to this beginners guide on Reiki where you will discover the amazing methods behind this great ancient practice from the east.

Reiki has been fascinating people for years and now you can learn these ancient methods within the next hour of reading this insightful guide.

I've wrote this short book in an easy to understand format so that you can easily apply what you learn fast all about Reiki and it's practices.

Keep an open mind and enjoy the spiritual journey.

Karen Hunt

# Chapter 1 – What exactly is Reiki?

In the last decades of human society development the spotlight has shifted towards finding alternative ways for healing and keeping balance in one's life. Stress and the speed at which we are required to perform or daily tasks transformed the way we live and look at things. In a considerable array of aspects, those changes had negatively impacted the quality of life and our ability to enjoy it.

Fortunately, we are living times in which modern physics is able to reveals what the ancients already knew. Our bodies are more than simple solid accumulations of matter.

Very powerful energy fields encompass our bodies, fluctuating according to our health, feelings and state of mind.

Although most of us are not able to see, evaluate or control this energy flow, there are a few who breached the barrier and are willing to help us enhance our understanding.

Reiki energy is a subtle kind of energy, very different than electricity or chemical energy or other kinds of physical energy you are normally aware of.

You could say that Reiki energy comes from the Higher Power, which exists in another dimension than the physical world we are familiar with.

Clairvoyants claim to see Reiki energy as coming down from above and entering the top of the practitioner's head, a place where the crown chakra reside. It then flows down through the body and out the hands.

Experienced practitioners are able to enhance the energetic flow and direct it mainly through their hands, where is mostly needed for healing practices applied to patient.

Many people fear to embrace Reiki practices because they fear it might interfere with their own beliefs system.

You have to understand that Reiki, although it involves a lot of spirituality and it addresses the concept of healing from within, is not a religion. Of course, like any other holistic practice, Reiki requires your full commitment and a strong belief in order to be effective and produce results.

Although it promotes the same core values of love and peace of mind, Reiki never tries to become a substitute for a given religion. A beginner in Reiki will never experience any restraints or contradictions in regard to the set of beliefs he/she was born with.

Reiki contains no dogmas, laws, prohibitions or conditions and gives total freedom to the individual. Reiki is nothing more than guidance towards becoming better and receiving more from life.

The term Reiki is obtained by combining two kanji (syllables). The first of them, REI, can be translated as universal, cosmic, and spiritual, while the second, KI, means power, strength and vitality.

By combining the two elements we are able to understand the essence behind Reiki and its claim to fame. By practicing Reiki you will be able to get in contact with the force that flows throughout the Universe.

Tuning yourself to its frequency means your body, mind and soul are welcomed to embrace new levels of development and harmony.

The vital force at the center of Reiki practices is not a new concept. Many ancient civilizations were able to sense its presence and highlight the benefits from getting in contact with it.

Called chi in China, barakka in India, ka in Egypt and pneuma in Greece, this cosmic force become in the era of modern science something more like a shadow.

It is worthy to know that mainstream scientist considers Reiki to be nothing more than the placebo effect. Nevertheless, many reported cases where people chose to believe and actually experienced a change to the better come as the perfect argument in favor of Reiki.

Reiki basically does most of its works at our mind level, by promoting five core principles of conduit. The five principles of Reiki are: today do not get angry, do not worry, be grateful, work diligently, and be kind to others.

## Chapter 2 – Reiki Initiation

Before proceeding any further the reader should know that Reiki is an evolving discipline, having many branches growing from the traditional Reiki developed a century ago.

In consequence there are many schools of Reiki claiming their own point of view on the initiation process. But beside the differences and tones, Reiki remains consistent in terms of core beliefs.

All ways of practicing Reiki target to connect our existence to the higher form of vital energy existing in the Universe.

It is very important to know from the beginning that Reiki is a discipline based on initiation. You can't claim be able to understand and practice Reiki by reading a book or by gathering theoretical knowledge from any other outside source. As the learning curve may become obstructed by the incapacity to evolve spiritually, the person in pursuit of initiation needs the guidance of a Reiki master.

Patience and taking things easy are also essential for embarking in the journey to become a Reiki initiate. Forget about fast results we are used from our speed-paced lifestyle.

Reiki is mostly about slowing down and concentrating on each step along the way.

The ability to access Reiki is conferred following a precise procedure called initiation, something that could be compared to a fine tuning, in which the teacher support its students to access the universal vital force.

Reiki Usui's method has two pillars: the daily practice of self-treatment (applying palms over different parts of your own body, in a certain order) and a daily conduit based on the five principles.

Each Reiki practitioner is initiated by a Reiki master, who was himself initiated and taught directly by another master Reiki, and so on, in an unbroken line, up towards Mikao Usui.

This process of initiation is taught only to those who reach the level of teacher / master. Other practitioners (Level 1 and level 2) are able to access Reiki but are not able to initiate someone else.

Initiation in Reiki cannot be done remotely and direct personal contact between the teacher and student should be made. The initiation procedure involves an information exchange at an energetic level.

It can be also considered to be a journey within and outside the self, a better understanding of its limits and shape. Because every person is unique, every session of initiation and every journey are also unique and personalized. A session is usually restricted to one hour, one hour and a half, depending of the level at which initiation is made.

Usui Reiki, also called traditional Reiki, has four degrees and each requires a separate approach on the initiation process. The fourth level is the level at which you can consider yourself to be a master.

This first level of Reiki has the role of making a short and superficial introduction to the energetic field that will later be explored. The vital energy is perceived at a coarse "resolution" and can be portrayed as a thin, invisible mist of water everywhere around us and inside ourselves. Students learn to communicate with the mineral, plant and animal kingdom using this energetic veil as a common denominator, able to minimize differences we would otherwise consider impossible to surpass.

Reiki is believed to be a universal language, glue for the fabric of the world. The established communication can take many forms, depending on the desired level (energetic, informational, and even spiritual).

After initiation for the first level of Reiki, the practitioner can do only self-treatment. In implementing self-treatment, hand positions are simple and intuitive. In principle, they travel from top to bottom, following the seven chakras, on the front and on rear of the body. Hands can also be applied on painful places.

After being initiated for the first level, the student receives the ability to activate its palms for a higher efficiency. The symbols of Reiki are also revealed to him. Reiki describes the symbols as keys able to unlock, modulate and amplify new levels of energy.

Level 2 of initiation allows the practitioner to remove negative energies from spaces and objects, purify crystals and energize water. At this level the initiated Reiki student is able to make extend its abilities beyond direct contact, making room for remote influencing. This is done mainly trough amplification and allows the creation of protection fields, which act as shields for any negative influences and could serve a house or person.

The second level helps us better know ourselves and better isolate the self. Connecting at this level provide an increase channel for the flowing energy to enter our system. Initiation for the second Reiki level is usually followed by an extended process of purification, for both the soul and the body.

Finishing the second level of Reiki initiation can be considered done when you get close to our true inner self and you become able to live in full consciousness. At this point you have full control over your emotions and you can chose to eliminate tension and worries.

Although Reiki initiation is usually done in the company of a master, from a certain point on, it's all left to you. You will need to win the battle between your old self and the new one emerging.

Reiki traditionally reserves the third level for the degree of master. But no anyone can truly reach the level and commitment and understanding neccssary lo become a master.

Beside all the courses and guides claiming to take you through all the stages in a record time, Reiki is about finding your true call. Not all Reiki initiates will hear that call well enough to become masters.

This level is usually reserved only for personality enhancement and the initiated entering the third stage of Reiki needs to teach others and confront their problems and blockages. Reiki, like any other holistic practice, is based on cyclicality and reciprocity.

The students are those who help the teacher adapt and perfection its techniques, allowing him to ultimately become a master. His methods should become general solutions for the problems of daily concern.

A Reiki master should never give factual solutions, the same way there is no perfect recipe on how to live. He is only committed to teach Reiki knowledge and live its life in terms with Reiki energy.

For a student wanting to benefit as much as possible from the Reiki learning experience, a few instructions could turn out to be very useful. First of all, try to delimit yourself from any disturbing concern and be fully present at the course.

The day should revolve around the few hours dedicated for the Reiki initiation. Allow plenty of time to arrive at your appointment without being in a hurry. It is always better to walk towards the location the Reiki session will take place and visualize that walk as part of your spiritual awakening, something close to a walkabout.

Always dress in the clothes you feel most comfortable in and leave behind any desire to impress. If you are targeting to get closer to your inner self, it is a good idea to allow your true personality at surface. Also, limit or completely eliminate vice and any form of excess towards your body and senses.

Reiki values include simplicity and living life at a slower, more profound pace. Waiting for Reiki lesson with enthusiasm and optimism is the best way to open your mind and heart.

Knowledge is always more easy to assimilate for those who do not fear or reject it. Reiki is not about clinching to performance and being competitive. Reiki is about cooperation and honesty, first towards your master and finally towards yourself.

If you have chosen to follow the initiation process expect to tear down some self-imposed limits and limiting beliefs. Again, this should not be seen in terms of competitiveness and progress, but more in terms of self-development, a growing that takes place inside and it's hard to be visible from the exterior.

## Chapter 3 – Reiki Breathing Techniques

We often ignore the simplest things in life and concentrate to put together elaborate plans and methods, only to be disappointed. Respiration is probably the most common activity of the human body, and we do it without thinking too much about it.

Reiki practices put respiration techniques back in the focus, giving us the possibility to benefit as much as possible from our interaction with the environment.

Respiration is a component of the energetic exchange between the organism and the environment. The oxygen we extract from the air is transported to each cell where it undergoes aerobic metabolism. Although we don't see air, we know it's there.

Air is the nature's greatest gift, the free food for our living engines. But each respiration brings much more than air inside our bodies. We also receive a little piece from the energetic flow of the vital force we previously talked about.

So if the respiration technique is incorrect, we lose not one but two benefits for our body's balance and well-being. Respiration is able to influence the nervous system, the level of concentration and memory. It is also our biggest gate for eliminating toxins, another reason for you to be interested in finding ways to improve your technique.

A large percent of the adult population uses chest respiration, which is a superficial technique, able to limit the amount of oxygen that the body receives with each inspiration. Deficiencies don't stop here, as chest respiration also drains much more energy in order to be performed. Those who use chest respiration need a lot more cycles of inspiration-expiration per minute and tend to be more nervous, stressed and superficial.

Reiki practice promotes abdominal respiration as a more powerful and useful tool for the human body. Using it enables the body to become more efficient with the resources it uses and also enhances the ability to access the vital energetic flow. In abdominal respiration, the abdomen enlarges towards the exterior, laterals and also towards the spine.

Being deeper, abdominal respiration is felt more strongly throughout the body, engaging many organs and tissues in a slow paced movement tuned at the perfect frequency.

Each breathe allow more oxygen to get in and more waste materials to be expelled. As a bonus, even more KI will get into the system, consistently improving our life.

Respiration from the abdomen is learned by following the steps described here. A sited position or lying completely horizontal, with the feet close together helps the body achieve the level of relaxation it needs.

The mind needs to follow the same patter, so any troubling thoughts should be brushed aside. This exercise should be welcome without the worry of failing and not doing things right.

The mind should be blocked from generating negative thoughts and only the body should be allowed to "speak".

One palm is put on the Hara spot, one inch below the belly button, and the other immediately above. Open the mouth and gently push inside the abdomen. Let the air out and count to 6.

Allow a pause between the expiration and inspiration by counting to 2. Let the air in and count to 3. Repeat the exercise until you will see that the lower hand moves at a higher amplitude than the higher one, signaling that your breathing movement has shifted towards the abdomen.

This exercise can adapted in terms of the numbers at which you need to count, but remember that process exhaling should always be twice as long as inhaling.

Abdominal respiration is like a return your childhood, a time when worries and concerns haven't entered the stage yet. The systems composing your body will notice the change and feel rejuvenated.

You will feel like something heavy was lifted off your chest and you are able to breathe again. Abdominal respiration, together with other practices common to Reiki initiation will help the body rejuvenate both in functions and anatomy.

New resources of joy and well-being will be at your disposal, allowing you to have a more fruitful life. Like with any other new techniques, learning how to breathe from the abdomen depends on the level and commitment and degree of repetition you can invest in it.

## Chapter 4 – The Benefits of Reiki

In standard Reiki treatment, energy flows from the practitioners hands into the patient's body. The patient is usually lying on a massage table but treatments can also be given while the person is seated or even standing.

The position is less important and all that matters is the state of relaxation that needs to be achieved before the treatment starts. The client remains fully clothed during Reiki sessions. The practitioner places her/his palms on or near the patient's body in a series of hand positions.

These include positions around the head and shoulders, the stomach, and feet. Other, more specific positions may target the road that links the seven chakras. Each position is held for a limited amount of time, depending on the energetic need the master discovers at each point.

The whole treatment usually lasts around an hour, but again, the master is the one to better tell. Reiki works by allowing the vital energy collected by the master to be transferred to the patient/initiate. The mechanism is hard to explained but it basically works by tuning the two bodies at the same frequency, allowing resonance to take place.

According to the laws of entropy that govern energetic transfer, energy will flow from areas where it is present in large quantities (the master's body) to the areas where a void of energy is present (the patient's body). This is the same way temperature equalize itself between two bodies of different readings, or the same way air reaches the same pressure in communicating volumes.

Reiki can be seen as healing force that enters the stage when belief in modern medicine and our ability to heal or balance life is eroded.

Reiki can prove to be effective for a broad category of problems affecting our existence. To start with, Reiki is able to reactivate our lost spiritually and can be used as a way to appreciate non-material possessions and be grateful for the life we live.

Constant exercise can help increase intuition, creativity, and logical thinking. Depression and other psychological conditions can see substantial improvement, up the point when compassion and respect for life are reestablished.

Reiki usually works by removing energetic bottlenecks and cleaning negative energetic residues. Unfortunate events, trauma and exposure to constant stress are all responsible for favoring the occurrence of such obstacles for the individual to naturally express itself.

Reiki alone does not heal, but it gives us the tools to access the vital energy contact was lost with. The body has a remarkable capacity to heal itself without external aid, if allowed. But the patience needs first to believe that the treatment will prove to be effective.

Extended medical research was able to reveal that the efficiency of medical treatments and surgical interventions is directly linked with the state of mind of the patient. To put it more clearly in words, the first step towards healing is to believe you can heal.

This is the point at which Reiki inserts its most important addition.

The way Reiki works is strictly linked with the seven chakras distributed along the human body. Each chakra is responsible for governing over the well being of one or more systems or organs of the human body.

Reiki channels the vital energy available outside our body trough a specific chakra, thus allowing it to be directed where the need is expressed. Although Reiki is able to reduce pain and discomfort, the way it works usually targets the cause and not the symptoms.

Reiki practice proves to be a very powerful tool for fighting addictions of all sorts. By quieting down the material body and welcoming relaxation exercises, the need for excess and destructive habits is also reduced.

The Reiki initiate learns to control the urges by accessing full control over his mind and thoughts. A negative habit is usually a thought that escapes beyond our barrier of logic and grows to the point of being performed on repeated occasions.

We usually feel bad for not being able to counteract this weakness and frustration only works to fuel the performed action. From a certain point on, we no longer feel remorse and we gradually lose control over our life.

Reiki is not a magical remedy for incurable conditions modern medicine is currently starring powerless.

Many Reiki schools make their claim to fame exactly on the contrary, but no hard scientific proof and statistic data was able to prove that. This is not an argument to exclude such patients from practicing Reiki. Holistic healing works by resolving the profound existentialist theme of suffering from such a condition. Reiki provide closure for those unable to accept their misfortune.

They will no longer blame themselves, the world or the written faith and learn to see their condition as an opportunity to grow spiritually and achieving a powerful awakening.

The Reiki master does not share the same practices with the modern psychologist, but they both work to approach the individual on a more personnel level. Being overwhelmed with acceptance and understanding, the patient goes beyond its condition and learns to see that there is life left beyond any problem.

## Conclusion On Your Reiki Journey

So now I have taken you on a journey into the world of Reiki, I really do hope this short insightful book will help give you a closer understanding the power of Reiki for beginners.

The next step is to take action on what you have learned today.

Finally, if you enjoyed this book, then I'd like to ask you for a favor, would you be kind enough to leave a review for this book on Amazon? It'd be greatly appreciated!

Enjoy your journey,

Karen Hunt